L

MW01120698

Vagus Nerve Exercises

A Simple & Step-By-Step Beginner's Guide to Unlock Your Natural Healing Power & Boost Your Vagal Tone | Relieve Anxiety, Depression, Inflammation, Chronic Illness & More

Zeph Hunter

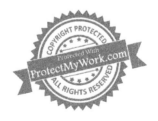

Table of Contents

INTRODUCTION

The vagus nervous system is considered to be one of the most vital nerves that are found in our body, but it is frequently overlooked when discussing well-being and health. This comprehensive guide is designed to improve that situation by offering an in-depth examination of the vagus nerve and its functions and the numerous methods and exercises that can be employed to boost its functioning.

The Vagus nerve is an extensive and wand-like nerve that runs through the brainstem, the thorax, the face, and down into the abdomen. The vagus nerve is by far the largest of cerebellar nerves and is responsible for controlling various bodily functions, such as heart rate, digestion, and immune system functions. It also plays an important role in regulating stress and emotional levels. The nerve is called"the "wandering nerve" because it travels through various organs and connects the brain to a myriad of systems within the body.

The advantages of improving vagus nerve functioning are many. Studies have shown that exercises for the vagus nerve and stimulation may help lower inflammation and improve the health of your heart as well as alleviate the symptoms of conditions like fibromyalgia and even help treat anxiety and depression. In addition, a functioning vagus nerve can be crucial for maintaining a healthy gut-brain connection, which is crucial for overall health.

Despite the many benefits of vagus nerve exercises people are not aware that they exist. This guide will make a difference by offering an extensive description of the vagus nerve and its various functions and also specific

instructions on how to perform different exercises and techniques for stimulation. We will also look into the most recent research about the relationship between the vagus nerve and a variety of ailments and will explore how these techniques and exercises can be utilized to improve the health of patients.

This guide was designed to be for readers of all levels of understanding and knowledge. It will start by explaining the fundamentals of the vagus nerve as well as its anatomy as well as physiology, and then go on to describe different stimulation techniques and exercises which can be employed to enhance the vagus nerve's function. We will also review the most recent research findings on the link between vagus nerves and various diseases and how these techniques and exercises could be utilized to improve the health of patients.

You may be a health professional who wants to broaden your understanding of the vagus nerve or a person looking to improve your health and overall well-being. This guide will give you the knowledge and tools that you require to harness the potential of the vagus nerve. At the end of this guide, you'll be more aware of the vagus nerve and the numerous ways you can boost its effectiveness to improve overall well-being and health.

CHAPTER 1:
WHAT IS THE VAGUS NERVE?

What happens when you go to Vegas is what stays in Vegas you think?

But the vagus nerve (pronounced as Las Vegas, the name that is Las Vegas), transmits signals to your heart, brain, lungs, and digestion system. It's the longest cranial nerve in your body, extending from your brain to the large digestive tract.

The vagus nervous system is considered to be one of the nerves that are most significantly found in our body, but it is frequently overlooked when discussing well-being and health. The vagus nerve is the role of managing involuntary motor and sensory functions such as your heartbeat, mood, speech, and the output of urine. It aids your body to switch between your flight or fight response and your parasympathetic in which you're more relaxed.

In this chapter, we'll take a deep look at the vagus nerveand its function, and the reason for its significance to our overall health and well-being.

ANATOMY AND PHYSIOLOGY OF VAGUS NERVE

The vagus nerve is the most extensive of the nerves in the brain. it is located in the brainstem. It stretches through the thorax and face and down into the abdomen. It is often called"the "wandering nerve" due to its wandering through various organs, linking the brain with a variety of systems within the body. The nerve is divided into two branches, one left and right, each of which is responsible for different functions. Vagus nerves are responsible for controlling various bodily functions, such as:

- Blood pressure and heart rate Vagus nerve play an important role in controlling blood pressure and heart rate by controlling the relaxation and contraction of heart muscles. It also regulates the flow of blood to organs and assists to maintain stable blood pressure.

- Digestive function and digestion: The vagus nerve is a vital role in the digestion process, controlling the muscles in the gut and regulating the release of digestive enzymes. Additionally, it regulates stomach acid production as well as the release of liver bile.

- Lung function and respiration The vagus nerve regulates the breathing muscles and is accountable for slowing the rate at which you breathe during times when you are at rest or in a state of relaxation.

- The function of the immune system The vagus nerve is responsible for how white blood cells are produced, as well as the release of inflammatory substances. It also plays an important role in controlling your immune system's response to infections and injury.

- Stress levels and emotions The vagus nerve is linked to the brain's emotional centers and plays an important role in the regulation of stress and emotions.

One of the primary roles of the vagus nerve involves regulating the parasympathetic nervous system which is responsible for reducing the body's functions as well as promoting a state of rest. This is different from the sympathetic nervous system which can trigger the "fight or flight" response during times of stress. The balance between these two systems is essential for keeping overall health and well-being A healthy vagus nerve is crucial to keeping the balance.

THE IMPORTANCE OF THE VAGUS NERVE

The vagus nerve, also known as the tenth cranial nerve, is one of the longest and most important nerves in the human body. It originates from the brainstem and travels through the neck, thorax, and abdomen, connecting to various organs and muscles along the way. The vagus nerve is often referred to as the "wandering nerve" due to its extensive reach throughout the body.

The vagus nerve is responsible for regulating many of the body's functions and has a significant impact on overall health and well-being. Some of the key functions of the vagus nerve include:

1. Heart Rate Regulation

The vagus nerve plays a crucial role in regulating heart rate. When the vagus nerve is activated, it sends signals to the heart to slow down, which results in a decrease in heart rate. This reduction in heart rate is important for maintaining cardiovascular health, reducing the risk of heart disease and other related conditions. A slower heart rate also helps to improve blood flow, ensuring that the body is receiving adequate oxygen and nutrients.

2. Respiratory Control

The vagus nerve is involved in regulating the respiratory system. It helps to control the rate and depth of breathing, ensuring that the body is receiving enough oxygen. When the vagus nerve is activated, it signals the body to slow down breathing and take deeper breaths, improving oxygenation and reducing the risk of respiratory problems such as asthma and chronic obstructive pulmonary disease (COPD).

3. Digestive System Regulation

The vagus nerve is responsible for regulating the digestive system. It helps to stimulate the digestive muscles, increasing the production of digestive juices and aiding in the digestion of food. The vagus nerve also helps to regulate the transit of food through the digestive system, reducing the risk of digestive problems such as constipation and diarrhea.

By improving digestive function, the vagus nerve also helps to prevent nutrient deficiencies, promoting overall health and well-being.

4. Immune System Regulation

The vagus nerve is involved in regulating the immune system. It helps to reduce inflammation in the body, reducing the risk of chronic diseases such as heart disease, arthritis, and type 2 diabetes. The vagus nerve also plays a role in the body's natural defense mechanisms, helping to protect against infections and illnesses. By improving immune function, the vagus nerve helps to promote overall health and well-being.

5. Stress and Anxiety Reduction

The vagus nerve is involved in regulating the body's stress response. When the vagus nerve is activated, it can reduce stress levels and reduce the symptoms of anxiety and depression. The vagus nerve works by signaling the release of certain hormones and neurotransmitters that help to calm the body and reduce the symptoms of stress and anxiety. By reducing stress levels, the vagus nerve can also improve sleep quality and reduce the risk of sleep-related disorders such as insomnia.

In conclusion, each of the functions of the vagus nerve is critical for overall health and well-being. By maintaining optimal vagus nerve function, individuals can reduce the risk of various health problems and improve overall quality of life. Incorporating exercises that stimulate the vagus nerve can help to improve its function and enhance overall health.

CHAPTER 2:
DISEASES OF THE VAGUS NERVE AND RECOGNIZING SYMPTOMS OF INFLAMMATION

Vagus nerves play an essential function in controlling numerous body functions. However, despite its importance, the vagus nerve can become damaged or compromised, leading to various health problems. These problems can range from mild and manageable to serious and debilitating, affecting an individual's quality of life. Any dysfunction or irritation of this nerve could result in a myriad of health problems.

In this chapter, we will take a closer look at the diseases and disorders associated with the vagus nerve, exploring the causes, symptoms, and treatments available. Whether you are a healthcare professional, or someone looking to learn more about the importance of this critical nerve, this chapter will provide you with a comprehensive understanding of the diseases of the vagus nerve.

We will delve into conditions such as vagus nerve damage, vagus nerve disorders, and conditions such as gastroparesis, chronic obstructive pulmonary disease (COPD), and heart disease, all of which are associated with the vagus nerve. By the end of this chapter, you will have a better understanding of how the vagus nerve plays a critical role in overall health, and how to recognize and treat the diseases and disorders associated with it.

So, if you are ready to expand your knowledge and understanding of the vagus nerve and its associated diseases and disorders, let's get started!

DISEASES OF THE VAGUS NERVE

Many ailments and diseases can impact the vagus nervous system, leading to dysfunction. The most frequent are:

1. Vagus Nerve Damage

Vagus nerve damage is a condition in which the vagus nerve is damaged or becomes compromised, leading to a range of symptoms and health problems. Causes of vagus nerve damage can include physical injury, surgery, tumors, infections, and autoimmune diseases. Symptoms of vagus nerve damage can include digestive problems such as constipation and diarrhea, respiratory difficulties, heart rate irregularities, and difficulty swallowing.

In severe cases, vagus nerve damage can lead to life-threatening complications such as heart failure and respiratory arrest.

2. Gastroparesis

Gastroparesis is a condition in which the muscles in the stomach are unable to properly contract, causing food to remain in the stomach for an extended period of time. This condition is often associated with the vagus nerve, as the nerve helps to regulate the muscles in the stomach. Symptoms of gastroparesis can include nausea, vomiting, abdominal pain, bloating, and weight loss. Treatment for gastroparesis may include medications, dietary changes, and in severe cases, surgery.

3. Chronic Obstructive Pulmonary Disease (COPD)

Chronic Obstructive Pulmonary Disease (COPD) is a lung condition that causes breathing difficulties and can lead to respiratory failure. The vagus nerve plays a role in regulating the respiratory system and can become damaged in individuals with COPD, leading to breathing difficulties and other associated symptoms. Symptoms of COPD can include shortness of breath, wheezing, coughing, and fatigue. Treatment for COPD may include medications, oxygen therapy, and lifestyle changes.

4. Heart Disease

Heart disease is a condition in which the heart becomes damaged or diseased, leading to a range of cardiovascular problems. The vagus nerve is involved in regulating heart rate, and when the nerve becomes damaged or compromised, it can lead to heart rate irregularities and other cardiovascular problems. Symptoms of heart disease can include chest pain, shortness of breath, heart palpitations, and fatigue. Treatment for heart disease may include medications, lifestyle changes, and in severe cases, surgery.

5. Inflammatory Bowel Disease (IBD)

Inflammatory Bowel Disease (IBD) is a condition in which the digestive system becomes inflamed, leading to a range of digestive problems. The vagus nerve plays a role in regulating the digestive system, and when the nerve becomes damaged or compromised, it can lead to digestive problems such as constipation and diarrhea. Symptoms of IBD can include abdominal pain, bloating, and changes in bowel habits.

Treatment for IBD may include medications, dietary changes, and in severe cases, surgery.

6. Depression and Anxiety

Depression and anxiety are mental health conditions that can affect an individual's mood and well-being. The vagus nerve is involved in regulating the body's stress response and can become damaged or compromised in individuals with depression or anxiety. Symptoms of depression and anxiety can include feelings of sadness, irritability, and worry. Treatment for depression and anxiety may include therapy, medication, and lifestyle changes.

7. Multiple Sclerosis (MS)

Multiple Sclerosis (MS) is a chronic autoimmune disease that affects the central nervous system. The vagus nerve is involved in regulating the immune system and can become damaged or compromised in individuals with MS. Symptoms of MS can include muscle weakness, difficulty with coordination and balance, and vision problems. Treatment for MS may include medications, physical therapy, and lifestyle changes.

8. Post-Traumatic Stress Disorder (PTSD)

Post-Traumatic Stress Disorder (PTSD) is a mental health condition that can develop after an individual experiences a traumatic event. The vagus nerve is involved in regulating stress levels and can become damaged or compromised in individuals with PTSD. Symptoms of PTSD can include flashbacks, nightmares, and feelings of anxiety and irritability. Treatment for PTSD may include therapy, medication, and lifestyle changes.

9. Chronic Fatigue Syndrome (CFS)

Chronic Fatigue Syndrome (CFS) is a condition in which an individual experiences persistent and severe fatigue, even after rest and sleep. The vagus nerve is involved in regulating energy levels and can become damaged or compromised in individuals with CFS. Symptoms of CFS can include fatigue, muscle weakness, and difficulty concentrating. Treatment for CFS may include medication, lifestyle changes, and physical therapy.

10. Guillain-Barre Syndrome (GBS)

Guillain-Barre Syndrome (GBS) is a rare condition in which the body's immune system attacks the peripheral nerves. This can lead to muscle weakness and even paralysis. The vagus nerve can become damaged in individuals with GBS, leading to a range of symptoms including difficulty swallowing, abdominal pain, and changes in heart rate and blood pressure. Treatment for GBS typically involves immunoglobulin therapy, physical therapy, and lifestyle changes to help manage symptoms and reduce the risk of serious health problems. GBS can be a life-threatening condition, so early diagnosis and treatment are critical for optimal outcomes.

SYMPTOMS OF VAGUS INFLAMMATION NERVE

The vagus nerve is inflamed and can trigger a broad variety of symptoms, based on the part of the nerve which is affected. Common symptoms of vagus nerve irritation include:

1. Abdominal pain and discomfort

The vagus nerve plays a crucial role in regulating digestive function, and when it becomes inflamed, it can lead to abdominal pain, discomfort, and other digestive symptoms. Individuals may experience abdominal cramping, bloating, and changes in bowel habits, such as constipation or diarrhea. The abdominal pain can be sharp, dull, or aching, and may be accompanied by nausea or vomiting. These symptoms can be especially debilitating and can interfere with daily activities, so prompt diagnosis and treatment are essential for managing symptoms and improving overall health and well-being.

2. Difficulty swallowing

The vagus nerve is also involved in regulating swallowing, and when it becomes inflamed, it can cause difficulty swallowing, choking, and other symptoms. This can be a serious and potentially life-threatening condition, especially in older adults who are more susceptible to choking and other digestive problems. Individuals may experience difficulty swallowing liquids, solids, or both, and may even choke on their food or liquids. This can cause discomfort, anxiety, and even malnutrition, so prompt diagnosis and treatment are critical for managing symptoms and reducing the risk of serious health problems.

3. Changes in heart rate and blood pressure

The vagus nerve is involved in regulating the heart and blood pressure, and when it becomes inflamed, it can cause changes in heart rate and blood pressure. This can lead to dizziness, lightheadedness, and even fainting, which can be especially serious in individuals with pre-existing heart conditions or other health problems. Individuals may also experience changes in blood pressure, such as high blood pressure or low blood pressure, and changes in heart rate, such as tachycardia or bradycardia. These symptoms can be accompanied by chest pain, shortness of breath, or other cardiac symptoms, and can be life-threatening if left untreated, so prompt diagnosis and treatment are essential for managing symptoms and reducing the risk of serious health problems.

4. Breathlessness and wheezing

The vagus nerve plays a role in regulating breathing, and when it becomes inflamed, it can cause breathlessness, wheezing, and other respiratory symptoms. This can be especially serious in individuals with chronic respiratory conditions such as asthma or chronic obstructive pulmonary disease (COPD), as these conditions can already make breathing difficult. Individuals with vagus nerve inflammation may experience shortness of breath, especially during physical activity, and may develop a persistent cough or wheezing. These symptoms can be debilitating and can interfere with daily activities, so prompt diagnosis and treatment are essential for managing symptoms and reducing the risk of serious health problems.

5. Hoarseness and voice changes

The vagus nerve is also involved in regulating voice and speech, and when it becomes inflamed, it can cause hoarseness, voice changes, and other speech difficulties. Individuals may experience a change in the quality of their voice, such as a loss of volume or pitch, and may develop a persistent hoarse or raspy voice. This can make speaking and communicating difficult, and can also lead to social and psychological stress. These symptoms can be especially serious for individuals who rely on their voice for work or other important activities, so prompt diagnosis and treatment are essential for managing symptoms and improving overall health and well-being.

In addition to these symptoms, individuals with vagus nerve inflammation may also experience fatigue, muscle weakness, and changes in mood or mental health. The severity and duration of symptoms can vary, but prompt diagnosis and treatment are essential for managing symptoms and reducing the risk of serious health problems. Treatment for vagus nerve inflammation may include medication, physical therapy, and lifestyle changes to help reduce inflammation and improve overall health and well-being.

It's crucial to recognize that symptoms like this can be caused by a variety of conditions and are not always caused due to inflammation of the vagus nerve. An accurate diagnosis by a doctor is essential to identify the reason for the symptoms.

The recognition of signs of the vagus nerve is essential as early diagnosis and treatment can reduce the risk of more serious issues and improve overall health and well-being. If you experience one of these symptoms mentioned above, it is crucial to speak with a medical expert to identify the root of the problem and to receive the appropriate treatment.

In the following chapter, we will look at various stimulation and exercise techniques that can be utilized to improve the vagus nerve's function and decrease inflammation. In addition, we will look at the latest research regarding the relationship between vagus nerve function and various diseases and the ways these techniques and exercises can be utilized to improve the health of patients.

CHAPTER 3:
VAGUS NERVE EXERCISE

The vagus nervous system plays an essential part in regulating several of the body's functions. Any malfunction and inflammation in the nerve may cause a variety of health problems. In this chapter, we'll examine the reasons why vagus-nerve exercises are vital to maintaining overall health and well-being.

The vagus nervous system is accountable for controlling the parasympathetic nervous system which is responsible for slowing down the body's functions and encouraging a state of relaxation. This balance between the parasympathetic and sympathetic nervous systems is crucial to maintaining health and well-being. But, in modern-day life, many people suffer from constant stress and excessive activity in the sympathetic nervous system. This can lead to chronic inflammation and imbalance within the body.

The exercises for the vagus nerve are an easy and efficient method of improving the functioning of the nerve and help maintain an optimal balance between the parasympathetic and the sympathetic nervous systems. The exercises can be utilized to decrease inflammation, enhance the health of your heart, ease symptoms of ailments like fibromyalgia, and can even help combat anxiety and depression.

Vagus nerve exercises may aid in improving gut health and maintaining a healthy gut-brain connection. The brain and the gut are in close contact and the condition of the gut could affect mental well-being and health. Gut health is vital to ensure proper digestion, nutrient absorption, as well as overall immunity.

In addition, studies have shown that exercises for the vagus nerve can help improve immunity by regulating the creation of white blood cells as well as inducing the release of anti-inflammatory substances. This could help prevent and treat chronic diseases.

Vagus nerve exercises are simple to carry out and can be integrated into daily activities. They involve activities like deep breathing and meditation, yoga and singing, humming, and even laughing. These exercises can be performed at any time and any location, which makes them an easy and convenient option to boost vagus nerve functioning and general health.

In the end, vagus nerve exercises are an essential method to ensure general health and well-being. They can be utilized to lower inflammation, boost the health of your heart, ease symptoms of diseases like fibromyalgia, and can even help manage anxiety and depression. They also aid in improving digestion and maintaining a healthy brain-gut connection and enhancing immunity.

Implementing vagus-related exercises into everyday life could significantly impact overall well-being and health.

TYPES OF VAGUS NERVE EXERCISES AND HOW TO DO THEM

The exercises for the vagus nerve are a straightforward and effective way to increase the functions of the nerve and help promote an equilibrium between the parasympathetic and sympathetic nervous systems. Let's examine the various types of exercises for the vagus nerve, and offer guidelines on how to do these exercises.

1. **Deep Breathing** is among the most simple and effective vagus exercises for the nerve.

It is the practice of breathing slowly, deeply through the nose, then out with the tongue.

Deep breathing exercises can activate the vagus nerve, increasing the oxygen levels within the body. It also slows the heart rate which creates a state of relaxation.

To complete this exercise, you must sit in a comfortable posture with a straight back with hands placed on your stomach. Inhale slowly through your nostrils and feel your stomach rise as your lungs fill with air. Take a breath briefly then exhale slowly out of your mouth and feel your stomach drop as your lungs empty. Repeat the exercise for 5-10 minutes at least a few times per day.

There is a variety of deep breathing techniques that can stimulate the vagus nerve. A popular technique is the 4-7-8 breathing method which involves breathing in for four seconds while holding the breath for 7 seconds and then breathing out for eight seconds.

This technique can help reduce the rate of breathing and encourages a state of relaxation.

Another variant is diaphragmatic breathing which requires breathing deep into the diaphragm rather than shallowly into your chest. For diaphragmatic breathing, put the palm of your hand over your stomach, and the other one on your chest. Breathe deeply through your nose, filling up your stomach with air. Finally, exhale out of your mouth. This will push air out of your stomach.

It is essential to do regular deep breathing exercises to help create a habit. It's equally important to find an area that is quiet and comfortable for the exercise and ensure that you breathe slowly and deeply.

Incorporating deep breathing exercises into your daily life could have a major impact on your overall wellbeing and well-being. It helps lower stress levels, boosts mood, decreases blood pressure, and encourages relaxation. Regular exercise in deep breathing will help improve vagus nerve function as well as enhance overall health.

2. **Humming:** It is an efficient vagus nerve exercise that can be performed anywhere anytime, anyplace. It is the act of making a humming sound when exhaling to activate the nerve. It creates vibrations within the face and skull that trigger nerve endings of the larynx and pharynx and sinuses. They stimulate the vagus nerve.

For this exercise, you must sit or sit in a comfortable place and exhale out of your mouth while creating a humming sound. You can make any sound you like or even just an easy "mmm" as well as "nnn" noise. It's crucial to find the right volume and pitch that you like. You can repeat this exercise for a couple of minutes often throughout the day.

It is possible to hum when doing other tasks, like cleaning, walking, or even working. It is also possible to incorporate it into a yoga or meditation routine, which makes it easier to incorporate into your daily routine.

The act of humming can reduce anxiety, improve mood and encourage relaxation. In addition, it helps in improving breathing and enhances vocal cord performance, and increases general relaxation. It is also believed to aid sleep, increase immunity, and decrease symptoms of depression and anxiety.

It's crucial to keep in mind that humming exercises must be done with care when you suffer from excessive blood pressure or ear infections or sinusitis. You should always talk to your doctor before starting any new exercise program.

Integrating humming exercises into your daily life could have a major effect on overall health and well-being. It may help increase vagus nerve activity as well as reduce stress levels and encourage relaxation. Regularly performing music exercises can boost overall health and well-being.

3. **Singing:** The act of singing is an excellent method to stimulate the vagus nerve. It requires using the entire voice cords which aid in activating the nerve. Singing can activate the vagus nerve which can in turn assist in lowering blood pressure, and heart rate and improve relaxation.

To do this exercise, select an instrumental that you like and perform it at the top of the croon. It is essential to make use of the entire range and volume of your vocal cords and to sing with intent and emotion. Repetition this exercise for a short time often throughout the day.

Singing is a great activity to do alone or in a group like the form of a choir or singing group. It is also possible to incorporate it into yoga or meditation exercises, making it simple to incorporate into everyday life.

Singing is known to increase your breathing, lower stress, enhance well-being and emotional health, and can even decrease blood pressure. It also assists in strengthening the immune system as well as improving emotional and mental well-being.

It's crucial to keep in mind that singing exercises must be handled with caution when you suffer from voice issues and/or high blood pressure and you must always speak with your physician before embarking on any new exercise regimen.

Integrating singing into your everyday life could significantly impact overall health and well-being. It helps enhance vagus nerve functioning to reduce stress and increase relaxation. Regularly performing singing exercises will help enhance overall health and well-being.

4. **Yoga** The practice of yoga is a fantastic way to enhance the vagus nerve's function. Certain yoga poses, such as the downward-facing dog child's pose, as well as the corpse pose can help stimulate the nerves and aid in relaxation.

Downward-Facing Dog: This posture involves bending into an inverted "V" shape with your feet and hands placed on the floor. This posture helps stimulate the vagus nerve by increasing the flow of blood to your head and reversing how gravity affects the body. Practice, this posture begins on your knees and hands, by placing your wrists right beneath your shoulders, and your knees underneath your hips. Then, lift your hips upwards and back, bending your legs and arms, and then press your heels toward the floor. Keep this posture for 30 to a minute, then repeat the posture several times.

- **Child's Pose:** This is a resting posture that can help stretch the spine as well as stimulate the vagus nervous system. To practice this posture start by placing your knees and hands as you sit back on your heels, and then stretch your arms inwards. Let your head relax and let the tension go from your body. Do this for 30 to 60 seconds then repeat the posture several times.

- **Pose of the corpse:** This pose is an energizing pose that assists to stimulate the vagus nerve through relaxing and reducing stress. To practice, this posture lies on your back with your legs and arms stretched outand close your eyes. Breathe deeply and let your body let go completely. Do this for 5-10 minutesand then continue to do the same pose several times.

It's vital to keep in mind that while doing this type of exercise, it's recommended to begin slowly and gradually progress into the exercises gradually. The exercises aren't suggested for people suffering from certain medical conditions. It's always recommended to speak with a medical professional before starting any new exercise regimen.

5. **Cold exposure** : Exposure to cold like taking cold showers or bathing in cold water, may cause vagus neuron stimulation. This is due to the role of the nerve in regulating the body's reaction to temperature fluctuations. Cold exposure can stimulate the vagus nerve which can in turn assist in reducing blood pressure, and heart rate and induce relaxation.

To do this exercise, begin by showering warm and then gradually reducing the temperature until it is cold. You should remain in the cold water for between 30 and an hour, and then repeat the exercise for several rounds. It's best to start with shorter durations, and gradually increase the duration when you're used to it.

You can also do cold exposure by submerging yourself in cold water, such as rivers, lakes, or even the cold plunge pool. It is important to remember that this activity must be handled with care and you should consult your physician before beginning particularly if you suffer from any medical condition that could be affected by exposure to cold.

The benefits of cold exposure are known to boost circulation, improve your immune system improve mood and energy levels as well as aid in losing weight. It also aids in reducing inflammation as well as improves the health of your cardiovascular system and encourages relaxation.

The inclusion of cold exposure into your daily life could have a profound effect on health overall and well-being. It may help enhance vagus nerve functioning as well as reduce stress levels and encourage relaxation. Regular exposure to the cold will improve your overall health and well-being.

6. **Laughter** is proven to stimulate the vagus nerve and has been proven to be a useful instrument for reducing stress as well as encouraging relaxation. Laughing can trigger an increase in endorphins. They are the body's natural chemical that makes you feel good that help to create feelings of well-being and calm.

To do this take a look at a comedy or read a funny book or have a chat with your family and friends that can make you laugh. It is important to choose something that truly brings you to laughter. Repeat this routine for a short time often throughout the day.

Laughter has been proven to boost cardiovascular health, ease stress and boost mood. It also helps improve immunity. It can also help improve sleep, ease pain, and boost a sense of well-being.

Incorporating laughter into everyday life could have a major impact on your overall health and well-being. It may help increase vagus nerve activity and reduce stress, as well as promote relaxation. Regular practice of laughter can boost overall health and well-being.

It's crucial to keep in mind that laughing exercises should be handled with caution in the event of medical conditions. And you must always talk to your physician before beginning any exercise program.

THE EFFECTS OF VAGUS NERVE EXERCISES ON DEPRESSION AND ANXIETY

Anxiety and depression are common mental health issues that have an impact on the overall health of an individual. Vagus nerves play an important function in controlling the body's response to stress. It can be targeted by exercises that can help alleviate the symptoms of anxiety and depression.

Research has shown that stimulating the vagus nerve with exercises like deep breathing, humming as well as yoga, can help decrease symptoms of depression as well as anxiety. Exercises that focus on breathing deeply, specifically have been proven to stimulate the vagus nervous system and increase relaxation, which could reduce feelings of depression and anxiety. Singing, humming, and exposure to cold have been proven effective at stimulating the vagus nerve while decreasing symptoms of anxiety and depression. Here are some of the key effects of vagus nerve exercises on anxiety and depression:

1. Reduces stress and anxiety

Vagus nerve exercises have been shown to reduce stress and anxiety by increasing the activity of the vagus nerve. This in turn helps to regulate the body's stress response and improve overall mood and well-being. By engaging in regular exercise of the vagus nerve, individuals can reduce symptoms of anxiety and depression, such as worry, nervousness, and irritability.

2. Improves mood and mental clarity

Vagus nerve exercises have also been shown to improve mood and mental clarity. This is because regular exercise of the vagus nerve can help regulate the body's response to stress and improve overall mental and emotional well-being. Individuals who engage in regular vagus nerve exercises may experience increased energy, improved concentration, and better sleep, which can all contribute to improved mood and mental clarity.

3. Promotes relaxation and decreases symptoms of depression

Vagus nerve exercises have been shown to promote relaxation and decrease symptoms of depression. This is because the vagus nerve is involved in regulating the body's response to stress and anxiety, and regular exercise of the vagus nerve can help improve overall mood and well-being. By engaging in regular vagus nerve exercises, individuals can reduce symptoms of depression, such as fatigue, hopelessness, and apathy.

4. Increases resilience to stress

Vagus nerve exercises have also been shown to increase resilience to stress. This is because regular exercise of the vagus nerve can help regulate the body's response to stress and improve overall mental and emotional well-being. By engaging in regular vagus nerve exercises, individuals can become more resilient to stress, which can improve their overall mental and emotional well-being.

In conclusion, regular exercise of the vagus nerve can have a positive effect on anxiety and depression. By reducing stress and anxiety, improving mood and mental clarity, promoting relaxation, and increasing resilience to stress, vagus nerve exercises can help improve overall mental and emotional well-being. Whether done as part of a larger exercise program or as a standalone activity, vagus nerve exercises can be an effective way to manage anxiety and depression and improve overall health and well-being.

However, It is important to remember that these exercises must be carried out with caution in the event of specific medical conditions. Also, it is always recommended to talk with your physician before beginning any exercise program. It is also crucial to pay attention to your body and avoid pushing yourself to the limit. Begin by doing short sessions and gradually increase your time until you are comfortable with it.

Integrating vagus nerve exercises into your daily routine can result in decreasing symptoms of anxiety and depression. These exercises, as well as other exercises for the vagus nerve, can aid in improving the functioning of the nerve, and also promote an equilibrium between the parasympathetic and sympathetic nervous systems. Regularly practicing these exercises can enhance overall health and well-being.

This chapter covered the various vagus nerve exercises as well as instructions on how to execute these exercises. These exercises, which include slow breathing, deep breathing yoga, cold exposure, and laughing, can be easy and effective methods for improving vagus nerve function and help maintain an optimal balance between the parasympathetic and sympathetic nervous systems. These exercises have been found to have a profound impact on health overall and well-being, including decreasing anxiety and boosting mood, encouraging relaxation, increasing the immune system as well as treating specific ailments. It is essential to perform regularly and seek out a medical professional before beginning any exercise program. Integrating these exercises into your daily life could be beneficial to overall health and well-being.

CHAPTER 4:
YOGA AND VAGUS NERVE

In the previous chapter, we reviewed the many exercises that are able for stimulating the vagus nervous system. While yoga was not on the list, its effect on stimulating the vagus nervous system is such that it warrants a separate chapter. Yoga is a unique combination of physical poses along with deep breathing and meditation, provides an all-encompassing approach to well-being and health, and its ability to stimulate the vagus nerve is evident. In this section, we'll examine the profound effect of yoga on the vagus nervous system and the ways that regular practice can improve the overall health of your body and mind.

Yoga is a practice that has been in use for many thousands of years and is widely accepted as a beneficial form of exercise for the body and mind. It is known to increase endurance as well as strength, balance, and overall well-being. Recent research has revealed that yoga is effective in stimulating the vagus nerve which is responsible for controlling many different body functions.

Vagus is one of the longest that runs through the body, and it runs from the brainstem to the abdomen. It plays an important role in controlling the body's stress response and also controls the cardiovascular, digestive, as well as immune system. When the vagus nerve gets stimulated, it may help to decrease inflammation, improve the health of your heart, and can even alleviate symptoms of anxiety and depression. Studies have also demonstrated that those who have a vagal tone that is high (meaning vagus nerves are in greater activity) have a lower chance to be suffering from chronic inflammation and high blood pressure and even heart disease.

Yoga is a great method to stimulate the vagus nerve as it integrates physical exercises with meditation, deep breaths, and breathing. Asanas or postures are a great way to strengthen and stretch the muscles. Meditation and deep breathing can help calm the mind and ease stress. This combination of components allows for a holistic approach to well-being and health.

One of the most effective yoga poses for the stimulation of vagus nerves is "child's posture." The posture requires you to sit back on your feet and put your forehead on the floor while stretching your arms across in front of you. This posture helps stretch muscles in the shoulders and neck that can increase the flow of the vagus nerve. It also encourages relaxation and calmness by decreasing tension in the neck, head, and shoulders.

A different yoga pose that is effective to stimulate vagus nerves is the "camel posture." This pose involves kneeling on the ground, and then stretching your back while extending your hands toward your heels. This pose helps to stretch muscles in the neck and chest area and neck, as well as by stimulating the vagus nerve. This also facilitates greater breathing capacity by opening the chest and lungs.

Alongside these poses in addition to these postures, breathing exercises that are deep including "pranayama," can also help with stimulating the vagus nerve. A well-known pranayama method includes "alternate nostril breathing" which is the practice of breathing into one nostril, and then out via the opposite. This practice can help regulate nerves and decrease stress. It can also aid in stimulating the vagus nervous system. This also permits more relaxation by slowing breathing and reducing the amount of mental chatter.

Meditation is a different part of the practice that could aid vagus nerve stimulation. Concentrating on the present and getting rid of distractions can aid in reducing anxiety and stress. This could lead to an increase in the vagal tone. A study carried out by researchers at the University of Massachusetts found that regular meditation can boost vagal tone and increase heart rate variability which is a gauge of the vagal function.

Yoga has also a significant impact on the body's stress response. Yoga practice has been proven to lower the levels of cortisol stress hormone and boost your levels of the happy hormone serotonin. This may help reduce inflammation and increase a feeling of well-being.

One of the biggest advantages of yoga is the fact that it can be done for all ages and fitness levels. The practice can be altered to meet individual requirements and can be done in various settings regardless of whether in a yoga studio, in your home, or even at the workplace.

In the end, Yoga is an effective exercise to stimulate the vagus nerve. A combination of poses as well as deep breathing and meditation will help strengthen and stretch the muscles, relieve tension and stress, as well as encourage relaxation and calmness. Certain poses, like"camel pose" and "child's pose, "child's pose" as well as "camel pose" are particularly efficient in stimulating the vagus nervous system, and deep breathing exercises such as "pranayama" or meditation exercises. Regular yoga has been proven to lower levels of the stress hormone cortisol as well as increase levels of the happy hormone serotonin. It can also aid in reducing inflammation and improving overall health.

Integrating yoga into your daily fitness routine can significantly impact your mental and physical health especially if you're hoping to increase the vagus nerve. It's important to remember that you should consult your doctor or a certified yoga instructor before starting any new exercise regimen. If you follow the correct instructions and consistently practice yoga can be a potent method of stimulating the vagus nerve and enhancing overall health and overall well-being.

CHAPTER 5:
VAGUS NERVE MASSAGES

The vagus nerve is one of the longest and most important nerves in the human body. It extends from the brain, down through the neck, chest, and abdomen, connecting to various vital organs along the way. As a result, the vagus nerve plays a crucial role in regulating many of our body's functions, including heart rate, digestion, and even our emotional state. In recent years, there has been increasing interest in using vagus nerve massages as a way to improve health and well-being.

The purpose of this chapter is to explore the science behind vagus nerve massages and the different types of massages that are used to stimulate the vagus nerve. We will also discuss the benefits of vagus nerve massages, how to incorporate them into your routine, and some precautions and contraindications to keep in mind. By the end of this chapter, you should have a good understanding of what vagus nerve massages are, how they work, and how they can improve your health and well-being.

HOW VAGUS NERVE MASSAGES WORK

The vagus nerve, also known as the 10th cranial nerve, is a long, wandering nerve that originates in the brainstem and travels through the body, connecting the brain to many vital organs such as the heart, lungs, digestive system, and more. It is responsible for regulating a wide range of functions, including heart rate, digestion, and stress response.

Vagus nerve massages work by stimulating the vagus nerve and promoting the release of neurotransmitters and hormones that help to regulate the body's systems. The massage stimulates the nerve by applying pressure to specific points along its pathway, encouraging the release of these neurotransmitters and hormones and improving the overall functioning of the nerve.

In addition, vagus nerve massages also promote relaxation and stress reduction. The massage can help to lower cortisol levels (the hormone responsible for stress response) and increase the release of endorphins, which are natural painkillers and mood elevators. This reduction in stress and increase in relaxation can have a positive impact on a wide range of health conditions, including anxiety, depression, and chronic pain.

It is important to note that the effects of vagus nerve massages can vary greatly from person to person, and the specific benefits you experience may depend on several factors, including the severity of your condition, the length of time you have been experiencing symptoms, and the overall state of your health. However, incorporating vagus nerve massages into your routine can be a simple and effective way to support your overall health and well-being.

Whether you are looking to improve your immune function, digestive health, or reduce stress and anxiety, vagus nerve massages are a powerful tool that can help you to achieve your goals. With regular practice, you may begin to notice an improvement in your overall health and a reduction in symptoms related to a wide range of medical conditions.

TYPES OF VAGUS NERVE MASSAGES

There are several different types of vagus nerve massages that are used to stimulate the nerve. Some of the most common techniques include pressure point massage, acupuncture, and cranial nerve stimulation. Each of these techniques works in a slightly different way, but the goal is always the same: to stimulate the vagus nerve and improve its functioning. These include:

Pressure Point Massage

Pressure point massage involves applying gentle pressure to specific points along the vagus nerve. These points are typically located along the neck, chest, and abdomen, and can be easily located with the help of a practitioner. By applying pressure to these points, we can stimulate the vagus nerve and improve its functioning.

Vagus Nerve Massage for the Neck: This type of massage involves applying gentle pressure to specific points along the neck, which can help to stimulate the vagus nerve and promote relaxation.

Vagus Nerve Massage for the Ear: This type of massage involves applying gentle pressure to specific points along the ear, which can help to stimulate the vagus nerve and promote relaxation.

Vagus Nerve Massage for the Chest: This type of massage involves applying gentle pressure to specific points along the chest, which can help to stimulate the vagus nerve and promote relaxation.

Vagus Nerve Massage for the Abdomen: This type of massage involves applying gentle pressure to specific points along the abdomen, which can help to stimulate the vagus nerve and promote digestion.

Vagus Nerve Massage for the Face: This type of massage involves applying gentle pressure to specific points along the face, which can help to stimulate the vagus nerve and promote relaxation.

Each type of vagus nerve massage has its own specific benefits and techniques, and it is important to choose the type of massage that is right for you and your individual needs. With regular practice, you may begin to notice an improvement in your overall health and a reduction in symptoms related to a wide range of medical conditions.

It is important to note that while vagus nerve massages are generally safe and effective, they may not be appropriate for everyone. If you have a medical condition, it is important to talk to your doctor before incorporating vagus nerve massages into your routine to ensure that it is safe and appropriate for you. Additionally, if you experience any pain or discomfort during a vagus nerve massage, it is important to stop immediately and seek medical attention if necessary.

Acupuncture

Acupuncture is a type of traditional Chinese medicine that involves the insertion of thin, sterile needles into specific points along the body to stimulate the flow of energy, known as Qi. This flow of energy can help to promote healing and balance, and has been found to be an effective form of vagus nerve massage.

When applied to specific points along the neck, ear, and abdomen, acupuncture can help to stimulate the vagus nerve, reducing symptoms of anxiety and depression and promoting a sense of well-being. Additionally, acupuncture has been found to help improve digestive function and reduce symptoms of conditions such as IBS and GERD, which are often associated with vagus nerve dysfunction.

Acupuncture is a safe and non-invasive form of therapy that has been used for thousands of years to promote overall health and well-being. It is important to choose a qualified and experienced acupuncturist to ensure that you receive the best possible care and results.

It is important to note that while acupuncture is generally safe, it may not be appropriate for everyone. If you have a medical condition or are pregnant, it is important to talk to your doctor before incorporating acupuncture into your routine to ensure that it is safe and appropriate for you. Additionally, if you experience any pain or discomfort during an acupuncture session, it is important to stop immediately and seek medical attention if necessary.

Cranial Nerve Stimulation

Cranial nerve stimulation, also known as vagus nerve stimulation therapy, is a non-invasive form of therapy that uses electrical stimulation to activate the vagus nerve. This therapy has been found to be effective in reducing symptoms of anxiety and depression, as well as reducing symptoms of a range of medical conditions associated with vagus nerve dysfunction.

Cranial nerve stimulation therapy involves the use of a small device, similar to a pacemaker, that is implanted under the skin. This device delivers mild electrical impulses to the vagus nerve, helping to stimulate and improve its function.

The effects of cranial nerve stimulation therapy can be seen quickly, and many people report a reduction in symptoms within a matter of weeks. This therapy is generally safe and well-tolerated, and there are few side effects associated with its use.

It is important to note that cranial nerve stimulation therapy is not appropriate for everyone. If you have a medical condition, it is important to talk to your doctor before incorporating this therapy into your routine to ensure that it is safe and appropriate for you. Additionally, if you experience any pain or discomfort during a cranial nerve stimulation therapy session, it is important to stop immediately and seek medical attention if necessary.

BENEFITS OF VAGUS NERVE MASSAGES

Vagus nerve massages can offer a range of benefits to our health and well-being. Some of the most notable benefits include:

Reducing anxiety and depression: Studies have shown that vagus nerve stimulation therapy can help to reduce symptoms of anxiety and depression by promoting the release of neurotransmitters in the brain, such as serotonin and norepinephrine. These neurotransmitters are thought to play a role in regulating mood and reducing symptoms of anxiety and depression. Additionally, vagus nerve stimulation therapy has been shown to increase the activity of certain regions of the brain that are involved in regulating mood, further improving symptoms of anxiety and depression.

Improving digestive function: The vagus nerve plays a crucial role in regulating digestive function, and massaging this nerve can help to improve symptoms of conditions such as IBS and GERD. For example, massaging the vagus nerve can help to stimulate the production of digestive juices and enzymes, improving the absorption of nutrients from food. Additionally, massaging the vagus nerve can help to improve gut motility, reducing symptoms of constipation and diarrhea.

Reducing inflammation: The vagus nerve is involved in regulating inflammation throughout the body, and massaging this nerve can help to reduce inflammation. Inflammation is thought to play a role in the development of a number of chronic health conditions, including heart disease, stroke, and autoimmune diseases. By reducing inflammation, vagus nerve massages may help to reduce the risk of these conditions and improve overall health.

Improving heart health: The vagus nerve is involved in regulating heart rate and blood pressure, and massaging this nerve can help to improve heart health. For example, vagus nerve stimulation therapy has been shown to improve heart rate variability, which is a measure of how well the heart is functioning. Additionally, vagus nerve stimulation therapy has been shown to reduce the risk of conditions such as heart disease and stroke, as well as improving symptoms of conditions such as arrhythmias and hypertension.

Boosting immune function: The vagus nerve is also involved in regulating immune function, and massaging this nerve can help to boost immune function. This is thought to occur by increasing the activity of immune cells in the body, such as T-cells and natural killer cells, and by promoting the production of cytokines, which are molecules that play a role in regulating the immune response. By boosting immune function, vagus nerve massages may help to reduce the risk of infection and illness, and improve overall health.

Overall, vagus nerve massages are a safe and effective way to improve overall health and well-being, and can help to reduce symptoms of a range of medical conditions. If you are considering incorporating vagus nerve massages into your routine, it is important to talk to your doctor to ensure that this form of therapy is safe and appropriate for you.

In conclusion, the benefits of vagus nerve massages are many and varied, and can help to improve overall health and well-being by reducing symptoms of anxiety and depression, improving digestive function, reducing inflammation, improving heart health, and boosting immune function. If you are considering incorporating vagus nerve massages into your routine, it is important to talk to your doctor to ensure that this form of therapy is safe and appropriate for you.

HOW TO INCORPORATE VAGUS NERVE MASSAGES INTO YOUR ROUTINE

Vagus nerve massages can be incorporated into your routine in several ways, depending on your preferences and the type of massage you are interested in. Here are some tips for getting started:

Find a practitioner: If you are interested in pressure point massage, acupuncture, or cranial nerve stimulation, it is important to find a qualified practitioner who can guide you through the process. Look for practitioners who have experience working with the vagus nerve and are able to provide guidance and support.

Learn about self-massage techniques: If you are interested in self-massage techniques, there are many resources available online that can help you get started. You can also consider taking a course or workshop that focuses on vagus nerve massages.

Make time for massages: Incorporating vagus nerve massages into your routine can be as simple as setting aside time each day to practice self-massage techniques. Make sure you have a quiet, relaxing space where you can focus on the massage and allow yourself to be fully present in the moment.

Be patient: It can take time to see the full benefits of vagus nerve massages, so be patient and persistent in your practice. Remember, the goal is to stimulate the vagus nerve over time, so be consistent and persistent in your practice.

PRECAUTIONS AND CONTRAINDICATIONS

While vagus nerve massages are generally safe and well-tolerated, there are some precautions and contraindications to keep in mind. If you have a medical condition, it is important to talk to your doctor before incorporating vagus nerve massages into your routine. Here are some other things to keep in mind:

- Avoid massages if you have a fever or infection: Vagus nerve massages can stimulate the immune system, which can be dangerous if you have a fever or an active infection.
- Avoid massages if you have a heart condition: Vagus nerve massages can affect heart function, so it is important to talk to your doctor if you have a heart condition or take heart medications.
- Avoid massages if you are pregnant: Vagus nerve massages can affect hormone levels, so it is important to avoid massages during pregnancy.

In conclusion, vagus nerve massages are a powerful tool for improving our health and well-being. Whether you choose to work with a practitioner or practice self-massage techniques, incorporating vagus nerve massages into your routine can help you to feel more relaxed, reduce symptoms of depression and anxiety, and improve your overall health and well-being. So why not try incorporating vagus nerve massages into your routine today and see what benefits you can experience for yourself!

CHAPTER 6:
THE INFLUENCE OF FOOD ON THE VAGUS NERVE

Vagus nerves play an important function in controlling the body's response to stress, and in promoting relaxation. Foods we consume have an impact directly on the functioning of the vagus nerve. It could help improve or hinder its performance. In this chapter, we'll examine the impact of food choices on the vagus nerve as well as the foods that aid in its functioning.

Certain food items contain substances that help activate the vagus nerve, and encourage relaxation. This includes foods that are rich in omega-3 fats like flaxseed and fish. Omega-3s are anti-inflammatory and are believed to help improve the function that the vagus nerve performs as well as reduce stress.

Probiotics, which can be present in fermented foods such as yogurt and kefir can assist in supporting the vagus nerve. Probiotics are a great way to boost the health of your gut which can aid in improving the functioning of the vagus nerve.

Consuming foods that are high in antioxidants, like vegetables and fruits, may aid in supporting the vagus nerve. Antioxidants may help in reducing inflammation, which may help in enhancing the function of the nerve as well as promote relaxation.

Foods high in refined sugars as well as processed foods may negatively impact the vagus nerve. These foods may cause inflammation and adversely impact gut health, which could hinder the function of the nerve and cause stress.

In addition to the mentioned foods, eating spicy foods and herbs like turmeric, ginger, and black pepper may aid in activating the vagus nerve, and help promote relaxation.

It's crucial to keep in mind that these food items should be eaten in moderation, and should be included in an overall healthy diet. Get advice from a health expert or a certified practitioner before making any major adjustments to your food habits.

FOODS TO EAT
For specific food items to eat, we suggest:

- Omega-3-rich fatty acids from fish and various other food sources, such as flaxseed and Chia seeds
- Fermented foods like sauerkraut, yogurt, sauerkraut and Kimchi
- Vegetables and fruits that are rich in antioxidants, such as leaves, berries, and sweet potatoes
- Herbs and spicy foods like turmeric, ginger, and black pepper

FOODS TO AVOID
Some of the food items to stay clear of include:

- Refined and processed foods that are high in sugars added to them and saturated fats
- Fried food items

- Artificial sweeteners
- Excessive consumption of caffeine and alcohol

In the end, this chapter will discuss the impact of food items on the vagus nerve as well as the food items that help support its functions. Integrating these food items into your daily routine, in conjunction with other exercises for the vagus nerve, will help improve the functioning of the nerve and help to maintain an equilibrium between the parasympathetic and sympathetic nervous systems. Regularly performing these exercises can improve your overall health and well-being. It's crucial to remember that a balanced and healthy diet is crucial and it is always best to speak with a health expert or a certified practitioner before making any major modifications to your diet especially if you suffer from any medical condition. Consuming a diet high in probiotics, omega-3s, anti-oxidants, and spices will help activate the vagus nerve and encourage relaxation. Avoiding refined and processed food items, fried and processed food items, artificial sweeteners and excessive consumption of alcohol and caffeine will help improve the functioning of the nerve and decrease stress.

CHAPTER 7:
MANAGING STRESS AND THE VAGUS NERVE

Stress is a normal aspect of life, however, it can have a negative impact on both mental and physical well-being, with particular emphasis on the functioning of the vagus nerve. It is accountable for regulating the body's stress response, and when it's stressed this can cause various health issues. Chronic stress can result in the vagal tone being diminished and can cause numerous problems, such as digestive issues as well as respiratory problems, as well as an increased risk of developing chronic illnesses. We'll look at how stress impacts the vagus nerve, strategies to manage stress, and meditation and mindfulness techniques to improve vagus nerve health.

STRATEGIES FOR MANAGING STRESS

In the beginning, it's crucial to comprehend how stress impacts the vagus nerve. When your body is under tension, the sympathetic nervous system gets activated, which releases cortisol and adrenaline. These hormones are vital to activate the "fight or fight" response, however, when they release in response to prolonged stress, they may result in an overworked or overstimulated vagus nervous. This could result in an increase in vagal tone as well as an increased level of inflammation which could lead to various health issues.

One approach to control stress and improve vagus nerve health is by doing deep breathing exercises. Methods like pranayama, as well as diaphragmatic breathing, can help to stimulate the parasympathetic nervous system that is accountable for the "rest and digestresponse. This helps calm the mind and decrease stress levels, and promote overall relaxation and well-being.

Another way to manage stress is to practice meditation and mindfulness practices. Meditation and mindfulness can assist to ease stress and increase overall well-being by encouraging calm, reducing negative thoughts and feelings, and improving self-awareness. In addition, these techniques can aid in reducing inflammation and improving vagus nerve functioning.

It is important to remember that stress management can be different for each person and it's crucial to figure out what works best for you. Certain people get relief from exercise, however, others might find meditation or yoga more efficient. It's important to find an appropriate balance of activities that are relaxing as well as activities that are stimulating.

A STRESS MANAGEMENT TO INCREASE VAGUS NERVE HEALTH

Implementing stress management strategies in your daily routine could aid in improving your vagus nervous system function. This can decrease inflammation, and improve overall health and well-being. Although it's impossible to eliminate stress but taking care of it in a healthy way will help stop the condition from getting chronic and consequently, lower the chance of having a negative effect on the vagus nerve.

It is important to speak with the healthcare professional before beginning any new methods for stress management. They can assist you through the most effective strategies for managing stress as well as improving the health of your vagus nerve.

In the end, stress has an impact on the vagus nerve's function, however, with the proper techniques and consistent exercise, it's possible to control stress and improve the vagus nerve's health. By incorporating relaxation methods including mindfulness, meditation, and other practices into your routine, you will be able to lower stress levels, encourage relaxation and enhance general well-being. Always remember to speak with a medical professional before implementing any new techniques for managing stress.

CHAPTER 8:
PUTTING IT ALL TOGETHER

Inducing the vagus nerve to stimulate it can have a major impact on your overall health and well-being, however, it's crucial to recognize that there isn't an all-encompassing solution. In this section, we'll look at the importance of integrating several techniques to create the perfect vagus nerve stimulation program that incorporates lifestyle changes and ensures vagus nerve health. A comprehensive strategy for vagus stimulation that includes not just physical exercises, but also adjustments in diet and lifestyle will yield better and longer-lasting results.

SCREENING A PERSONALIZED VAGUS NERVE STIMULATION PLANNING

The first step to creating an individual vagus nerve stimulation program is to evaluate your current state. This involves assessing the current vagal activity, as well as identifying health issues, and then evaluating the stress levels you are currently experiencing. When you have a clear knowledge of your current state and your current situation, you can establish achievable and precise objectives for yourself. For example, if suffer from constant stress, you could establish a goal of reducing the stress level within a certain period.

The next step is to include different methods in your program. It could be a combination of deep breathing exercises as well as yoga as well as cold exposure, singing, and much more. It is essential to find the right balance of strategies that work for you and can integrate into your routine. Try different methods and determining what works best for you is crucial.

It's also crucial to track the progress of your mental and physical well-being. This can be accomplished by observing any changes in your symptoms or energy levels as well as overall health. This will help you identify which methods are the most efficient and adjust them whenever necessary. Continuously reviewing your progress can allow you to modify your strategy as needed to reach your goals.

INCORPORATING LIFESTYLE CHANGES

Alongside incorporating physical activities, it's crucial to implement lifestyle adjustments that promote the vagus nerve's health. Consuming a balanced diet rich in vegetables, and fruits, along with omega-3 fats could aid in reducing inflammation and improve overall health. Sleeping enough as well as decreasing stress levels, engaging regularly in physical exercise, and limiting exposure to toxic substances and toxins can all help support Vagus Nerve health. These adjustments not only improve vagus nerve health but also improve overall health and well-being.

MAINTAINING VAGUS NERVE HEALTH

Stimulating the vagus nervous system is a continuous process, and it's crucial to maintain regularity in your routine. This involves adding vagus nerve stimulation techniques into your schedule and making it part of your daily routine. Also, speaking with a medical professional before beginning any new vagus nerve stimulation technique will assist you in determining the best methods to meet your requirements, and also help keep track of the progress you make. It is crucial to be aware that results might not be immediate and to allow your body to adjust and adapt to the changes that you are creating.

In the end, stimulating the vagus nerve could be a major influence on general health and well-being. But, it's essential to keep in mind that a comprehensive approach is required to get the greatest outcomes. Utilizing a variety of techniques, developing your vagus nerve stimulation program as well as incorporating lifestyle changes, and ensuring consistency in your routine are all crucial actions to unlock the potential of the vagus nerve. Be sure to be aware of your body, remain patient, and make changes as necessary to ensure that you are in the right direction to achieve the best health of your vagus nerve.

CHAPTER 9:
PRECAUTIONS AND CAUTIONS

It is important to remember that the information contained in this book isn't meant to replace any advice from a medical professional. It is always recommended to speak with a medical professional or a qualified practitioner before beginning any exercise program or making major adjustments to your diet particularly if you suffer from any medical issues.

Certain individuals may have medical conditions that may cause certain food or exercise to be hazardous. For instance, those with blood pressure problems should avoid exercises that require keeping or lowering their breathing, like"Humming" or the "Humming" practice. Those with chronic respiratory ailments such as asthma must avoid exercises that require them to hold their breath, for example, breathing exercises like the "Breath and Holding" exercise. If you've had an antecedent history of heart disease it is important to talk with a medical professional before attempting exercising with the "Cold exposed" exercise.

It is important to pay attention to your body and don't overdo it. If you feel discomfort, pain, or other symptoms, stop your exercise and speak to an expert in healthcare. It is always recommended to begin with short periods and then gradually increase the amount of time when you're comfortable with it.

HOW TO TELL WHETHER THE EXERCISES ARE WORKING

It's crucial to evaluate the effectiveness of your exercises to see whether they're working and when it is time to seek medical assistance. Here are some indicators to look for:

- Better mood: You should start to notice improvements in your mood like being more relaxed and less stressed.
- Better sleep: You could discover that you're more comfortable sleeping and feel more refreshed when you wake up.
- Stress reduction: You will be able to notice a decrease in stress and an overall feeling of peace.
- Better digestion could notice that you're having less discomfort and bloating and your stool movements are becoming more regular.
- Immune function is improved You might notice that you're getting sick less frequently and the time to recover is less.

It's crucial to keep in mind that each person's experience is unique and it could take time before you can notice any improvement. It's also crucial to keep in mind that these exercises are part of a comprehensive method of improving your overall health and well-being. If you don't see any changes or if you notice your symptoms get worse it's crucial to talk to an expert in your healthcare for further assessment and guidance.

It is also important to note that the exercises in this book aren't meant to substitute for any medication or medical treatment recommended by a medical professional. If you're currently under medical treatment or taking medications, it's essential to talk to your doctor before beginning any new exercise routine or making significant adjustments to your eating habits.

In the final section, this chapter will discuss the importance of speaking with an experienced healthcare professional before starting any exercise routine or making significant changes to your diet and also how to evaluate the efficacy of exercises and know when to get medical advice. It is important to keep in mind that these exercises are an integral part of a holistic method of improving your overall health and well-being and should not be used as a substitute for any medication or medical treatment recommended by a medical professional.

CHAPTER 10: QUICK VAGUS NERVE EXERCISES

The vagus nerve can be a positive influence on overall health and well-being if it is working optimally. In today's fast-paced environment, however, the vagus nerve may become overstimulated, leading to anxiety, depression, chronic inflammation, and other health issues.

This chapter briefly lists easy exercises to improve the vagus nerve's quality. Each exercise targets specific areas of your body to enhance vagus nerve function. These exercises are easy to incorporate into busy lives and take only 30 minutes.

Deep breathing exercises (diaphragmatic breath)

Deep breathing, also called diaphragmatic or diaphragmatic breathing, can activate relaxation and stimulate the vagus nerve. Inhaling through your nose, filling your lungs with air, allowing your diaphragm and belly to expand, and then slowly exhaling through the mouth to let go of the air. This quick and simple technique can be used anywhere and at any time.

Steps:

- You can sit or lie down in a quiet area with your back straight. Your shoulders should be relaxed.

- One hand should be placed on your stomach, just below the rib cage. The other hand should be on your chest.
- Slowly inhale through your nose. Feel your belly expand while you fill your lungs. Your stomach should rise higher than your chest.
- For a few seconds, hold your breath and then exhale slowly through your mouth. As you release the air, your belly will begin to shrink. Your exhale should be longer than your inhale.
- For several minutes, focus on the sensation of your breathing moving in and out of your body. Let go of all distractions and thoughts.
- To increase your relaxation response, you can either gradually increase the length of the exhales or inhales or use guided meditation or visualization.

Tips:

- To establish a routine, practice deep breathing exercises every day for at least a few minutes, preferably in the same spot and at the same time.
- Deep breathing can occur while standing, sitting, walking, lying down, or standing.
- Avoid deep breathing and chest breathing. These can trigger the stress response in the body and create tension.
- Deep breathing exercises can be combined with other relaxation techniques like progressive muscle relaxation or visualization.

- Before you start any exercise or new wellness program, consult your healthcare professional, especially if there are any respiratory or cardiovascular conditions.

Yoga

Yoga is a mind and body practice that includes a variety of postures, breathing exercises, meditation, or relaxation techniques. Yoga has positively impacted the nervous system, including the vagus nerve. These are the steps for performing a simple yoga sequence.

Yoga Sequence:

- Find a quiet and comfortable place to practice. Comfortable clothing allows for movement.
- Start with a few deep breaths to calm the mind and prepare your body. You can sit cross-legged on a table or in a chair, with your back straightening and your hands on your knees. Take a deep inhale through your nose and close your eyes. For a few seconds, hold your breath and then slowly exhale through your mouth. Continue this for several minutes, paying attention to the sensation of your breath moving through your body.
- Begin by warming up with gentle stretches. Begin by standing straight up with your feet at your sides and arms extended. Exhale, and grow your arms overhead. Inhale, fold your arms forward, and reach your fingers toward your toes. After holding for a few seconds, inhale slowly and roll until standing.

- You can move into a series (or asanas) of yoga poses to stimulate the vagus nerve and promote relaxation. Some examples include:
- Dog facing downward: Begin on your hands and knees with your wrists below your shoulders and your knees beneath your hips. Inhale, lift your hips upwards, and create an inverted V shape with your body. If necessary, keep your knees bent and your heels off the ground. Take a few deep breaths and hold for a while. Then exhale and bring your knees back to your chest.
- Bridge pose: Place your hands on your hips and your feet flat on your floor. Exhale, lift your hips towards the ceiling, and press your shoulders and feet into the ground. Hold the position for a few seconds and then exhale to lower to the ground.
- Child's pose: Place your hands on your knees and your wrists below your shoulders. Keep your knees bent and your hips in line with your elbows. Inhale, and bring your hips down towards your heels. Stretch your arms out in front. Rest your forehead on the ground for a few seconds and take a deep breath.
- Legs up the wall: Lie on your left side before a wall. Your legs should be straight up against the wall. Your arms should be at your sides. For a few moments, relax and breathe deeply.
- End your meditation or relaxation session with a few moments of silence. Place your palms on the top of your head, and lie down on your back. Relax your body by closing your eyes. You can also do guided relaxation or visualization exercises to calm your mind and body.

Meditation

Meditation, a mindfulness-based practice, is about focusing on one object, thought, or sensation at the moment. Meditation has many health benefits, including improved mood, stress reduction, brain function, and stress management. These are the steps you need to take to start meditation.

- You will need to find a peaceful and quiet place to meditate.
- You can sit on a cushion or a chair, flatting your feet on the ground.
- Keep your eyes closed, or look down softly. Now, focus on your breath.
- Start to take slow, deep, slow breaths. Inhale through your nose, and exhale through your mouth.
- Pay attention to the sensations of your breath moving in and outside your body. Next, focus your attention on the feelings of your nostrils and the rising and falling sensations in your belly or chest.
- Your mind may wander if you are unable to focus on your breath.
- You can count your breaths or repeat a mantra or phrase to anchor your attention.
- Try to meditate for at least five to ten minutes per day. Gradually increase the time as you get more comfortable with the practice.

Regular meditation practice can help you cultivate calmness and inner stillness over time.

Chanting or Singing

Chanting or singing involves the use of vocal cords and a diaphragm. This can stimulate the vagus nerve and promote relaxation. Chanting and singing are often used in religious or spiritual practices. They can also have psychological and emotional benefits.

Steps:

- You can choose a song, chant, or other music that you like or that has a relaxing effect.
- You will need a private, quiet space to sing or chant.
- You can either stand straight up or lie down with your back straight and your feet flat.
- To center yourself and relax, take a few deep breaths.
- Start singing or chanting at an appropriate volume and pace.
- Concentrate on the sensations in your voice and vibrations within your body.
- Instead of relying on your vocal cords, use your diaphragm instead.
- You can sing or chant with others if you feel comfortable.
- Continue singing and chanting for as long as you feel comfortable.
- Take a few minutes to relax after you are done.

Tips:

- Try different music and chants to discover what resonates the most with you.

- You don't have to be perfect at singing or chanting - the goal is to enjoy the experience and feel the vibrations within your body.
- You may feel self-conscious singing or chanting. Try doing it with others to feel supported and connected.
- To make singing and chanting a habit, you can incorporate them into your daily life, such as during the morning shower or on your commute.

Cold exposure (cold water immersion, cold showers)

Cold exposure is when the body is exposed to cold temperatures. This can trigger the response of the sympathetic nervous system, the "fight or flight, " and the parasympathetic nervous system, the "rest and digest" response. You can cold expose yourself in a variety of ways.

These are the steps to perform cold exposure

- Begin slowly: If this is your first cold exposure, you can start by exposing for shorter periods and then gradually increase the exposure. Begin with a brief cold shower or a quick immersion in cold water.
- Preparing the body: Before you begin, take a few deep breaths and relax your body. Start with warm water, and slowly reduce the temperature to your desired temperature.
- Start by exposing your extremities to cold water. For cold showers, tell your feet and hands to use cold water. Next, move on toward the center of your body. You should stay in cold water immersion or a cold shower for no less than 30 seconds.

- Concentrate on your breath: This can calm your body and activate the parasympathetic nervous system, including the vagus nerve.
- Stop the exposure. Warm up slowly with warm clothing, blankets, or beverages after the exposure. Avoid taking a hot bath or shower immediately following cold exposure, as this could reduce the benefits.

Cold exposure is not recommended for everyone, especially those with certain medical conditions. To avoid injury or overexposure, consult a healthcare professional before you begin any exercise or wellness program.

Gargling with warm, saltwater

Warm salt water can gargle a sore throat or relieve a sore mouth. Saltwater is well-known for its anti-inflammatory and antibacterial properties and ability to fight bacteria and viruses.

These steps will help you perform gargling using warm salt water

- Mix 1/2 teaspoon salt in a glass of warm water. Stir the salt until it is fully dissolved.
- Take a sip and tilt your head slightly back.
- Allow the salt water to sit in your throat. Then, start gargling. Be sure to get the salt water into your throat. But be careful not to swallow it.
- Gargle for 30 seconds - 1 minute or until salt water runs out. Then, pour the salt water into the sink.
- To remove salt residue, rinse your mouth with water.

- You can repeat the process as many times as you need to get relief.

Gargling warm salt water with your mouth is not a substitute for medical treatment. It is important to remember that you should consult a healthcare professional if there are any concerns about your throat and mouth.

Laughter Therapy

Laughter therapy is also known as laughter yoga. It involves intentional laughter and can be used as a form of exercise. It is a way to reduce stress and improve well-being through laughter and breathing exercises. This is a step–by–step guide to performing laughter therapy.

- You should find a private, comfortable space to laugh freely without being judged or interrupted.
- Take a few deep breaths to help you relax your body and mind. Then exhale with a sigh.
- Begin with a fake, forced laugh such as "ha ha ha" and "hee, hee, hee," and then let it grow into contagious laughter.
- Use eye contact and body language even if you're laughing alone to increase laughter and build a sense of connection.
- Try out different types of laughter, such as silent and belly, and let your laughter flow without judgment.
- To increase oxygen flow to the brain and body, incorporate breathing exercises such as deep inhalation and exhalation with an "oh ho" sound.

- To help calm your mind and body, end the laughter session by taking a few minutes to slow down and deepen your breathing.

If you have any history of heart disease or other medical conditions, laughter therapy should not be used cautiously. It's always a good idea to consult a healthcare professional before starting any exercise or wellness program.

Vagal nerve stimulation therapy (using an implanted device).

VNS refers to a medical procedure that uses an implanted device to stimulate the vagus nerve. This long nerve runs from the brainstem to the abdomen. The FDA has approved this therapy for specific medical conditions such as depression and epilepsy. Some research has shown that VNS may benefit other health conditions, such as vagal tone enhancement.

Step-by-step procedure:

- Evaluation: You must undergo an extensive assessment to determine if you are a suitable candidate for VNS therapy. This could include a medical history review, a physical exam, or diagnostic tests.
- Implantation: The VNS device will be implanted if you are considered a good candidate. The VNS device is usually placed on the left side and connects to the vagus nerve in your neck.
- Programming: Once the device has been implanted, it must be programmed to provide the correct stimulation level. This is usually done by a healthcare professional such as an

epileptologist or neurologist. You can adjust the stimulus over time to maximize its therapeutic effects.

- Stimulation: After the device has been programmed, it will provide gentle electrical stimulation to the vagus nerve at regular intervals. You can adjust the frequency and intensity of stimulation as required.
- Monitoring: Your healthcare team will closely monitor you during VNS therapy to ensure your treatment is safe and effective. Regular follow-up visits, diagnostic tests, and adjustments to stimulation settings may be required.
- Lifestyle modifications: Your healthcare team may suggest lifestyle changes to improve the effectiveness of VNS therapy. These could include lifestyle changes such as exercise, stress reduction, and dietary modifications.

VNS therapy should only be used under the supervision of a qualified healthcare professional. Although it may benefit some medical conditions, it's not a panacea and may not suit everyone.

Cardiovascular exercises, such as running, swimming, or cycling, are physical activities.)

Cardiovascular exercises increase heart rate and work the cardiovascular system, including the heart and lungs. These exercises can improve your overall health and well-being, as well as the function of your vagus nerve.

Here are some steps to do cardiovascular exercises.

- Choose an activity: Pick an activity that increases your heart rate, such as swimming, running, cycling, or jumping. Choose an activity that you like and can do for at least 20 minutes.
- Warm up: Start with at least five minutes to prepare your body and muscles for exercise. You could do gentle stretching or light jogging.
- Begin your exercise by starting at a slow pace. Gradually increase the intensity of your workout as your body adapts. You should aim to exercise for between 20-30 minutes each session. However, this can be increased as your fitness level improves.
- You can monitor your heart rate by using a heart rate monitor. This is usually 60 to 80% of your maximum heartbeat, 220 times your age.
- Cool down: After your workout, take a few minutes to cool down. Slowly decrease the intensity of your exercises to get your heart rate back into resting mode.
- Stretch: After your cool-down, stretch your muscles to prevent injury and soreness. Each stretch should be held for between 20-30 seconds. Repeat the process 2-3 times.
- Hydrate: Keep hydrated before, during, and after exercise to maintain energy and hydration.
- Gradually increase intensity: As you get fitter, gradually increase the power of your cardiovascular exercises to keep your body challenged and to improve your fitness.

Notice: Before you start any exercise program, it's a good idea to consult with your healthcare professional.

Progressive muscle relaxation

Progressive muscle relaxation (PMR), a relaxation technique, involves relaxing and tensing specific muscle groups to relieve tension and stress. This technique can reduce anxiety and lower blood pressure. It also promotes relaxation and calmness.

Step-by-step procedure:

- You will need a place where you can relax and unwind.
- Take a few deep, slow inhalations. Inhale slowly through your nose. Exhale through your mouth.
- Begin by tensely clenching your toes and feet for 5-10 seconds. Next, let the tension go and relax the muscles for 15-20 seconds.
- Next, tighten your calves muscles and hold them for 5-10 seconds. Then release the tension and relax for 15-20 seconds.
- Begin to move up to your thighs and hold for 5-10 seconds before releasing for 15-20 seconds.
- Tend your stomach, chest, and back muscles one at a time. Hold for 5-10 seconds, then release and relax for 15-20 seconds.
- Now, move on to your upper arms and shoulders. Tend and hold for 5-10 seconds. Then relax for 15-20 seconds.
- Tend your lower arms and hands and hold for 5-10 seconds, then relax for 15-20 seconds.
- Next, relax your facial muscles and neck by tensing them for 5-10 seconds.
- Focus on your relaxation and take a few deep breaths.

- Depending on how stressed or tense you are, repeat the process as often as possible.

Tips:

- Throughout the exercise, take a deep and slow breaths.
- Concentrate on the differences between tension and relaxation in each muscle.
- You should do it regularly to improve your ability to practice PMR and reap its full benefits.
- While doing PMR, you can also use visualization techniques.
- Do not clench your muscles to the point that you feel pain or discomfort.

Acupuncture

Acupuncture, a traditional Chinese medicine practice, involves the incision of thin needles at specific points on the body to promote healing. It is believed that the method stimulates specific nerves, including the vagus. This improves blood flow and energy flow throughout your body.

These are the steps to perform acupuncture.

- You should find a licensed and accredited acupuncturist. You should look for someone licensed and certified to practice acupuncture.
- Consultation: The acupuncturist will conduct the consultation to review your medical history and discuss any health concerns. They may examine your pulse and tongue to determine the best treatment plan.

- The acupuncturist will create a treatment plan based on your consultation. This may include a series of sessions. The acupuncturist will determine which acupuncture points should be targeted and which could stimulate the vagus nerve.
- Needle insertion: The acupuncturist will place thin needles in specific points of your body during the treatment. The hands will remain in place for 20-30 minutes while you relax and lie still.
- Needle removal: The acupuncturist will safely dispose of the needles after the treatment. Mild soreness and bruising may occur at the insertion site, but it usually disappears quickly.
- Your acupuncturist may recommend additional treatments depending on your condition and response.

Acupuncture is not recommended for everyone. Licensed and certified professionals should only do it. Before you begin acupuncture, talking with your healthcare provider about any side effects or potential risks is important.

Massage Therapy

Massage therapy is a relaxing and effective way to stimulate your vagus nerve. There are many branches of the vagus nerve that run throughout the body. These include the stomach, neck, back, and back. Massage can be used to stimulate the nerves and promote relaxation. These steps will help you perform vagus nerve stimulation massage therapy:

- You can lie down on your back or in a chair that supports your back.
- To calm down and relax, take a few deep breaths.

- Start by making gentle circular movements on the sides and neck below your ears. Apply light pressure with your fingertips in a clockwise motion.
- Massage the neck area by moving down to the collarbone.
- Use gentle pressure to massage the middle of your sternum (breastbone) in a circular motion.
- Massage the stomach with gentle circular movements.
- Take a few deep, slow breaths. Then relax and feel the sensations throughout your body.

Massage therapy should only be done by trained professionals or under their supervision. Incorrect pressure or massage techniques can lead to injury. Massage therapy is unsuitable for all people, especially those with certain medical conditions. Before you start any exercise or wellness program, it's a good idea to consult with your healthcare provider.

Tai Chi and Qigong

Tai Chi and Qigong, ancient Chinese practices, combine breathing techniques with physical movements to improve physical and mental well-being. Anyone of any age and fitness level can do Tai Chi and Qigong. These exercises improve balance, flexibility, and coordination, reducing stress and encouraging relaxation.

Step-by-Step Guide:

- Start by standing straight up with your feet shoulder-width apart; your arms extended to your sides. Keep your back straight and relax your shoulders.

- Take a deep inhale through your nose and exhale through your mouth slowly. Focus on relaxing tension.
- Slowly lift your arms to shoulder height. Keep your elbows bent and your palms down.
- Your weight should be on your left foot. Now, lift your right foot off the ground by bending your knee. Your foot should be back on the ground.
- Step 4: Shift your weight to the right foot and repeat step 4.
- Continue to shift your weight from one foot towards the other, slowly and controlled.
- While shifting your weight from one foot to the other, lift your opposite arm to shoulder height. Keep your elbows bent and your palms down.
- Lower your foot to the ground and lower your arm to your side.
- For several minutes, focus on your breathing and keep a steady pace.
- Once you are comfortable with the basics, you can add complex sequences and movements to your practice.
- Slowly lower your arms to your sides and take a few deep breaths.

Tai Chi and Qigong require patience. Regular practice is necessary to reap the benefits. To ensure you do the exercises safely and correctly, it is a good idea to consult a qualified instructor before starting your practice.

Mindful Eating

Mindful eating is about paying attention to what you eat and focusing on the texture and taste of the food. It also involves being present while eating. Mindful eating can improve digestion and prevent overeating. It also promotes a better relationship with food.

Here are some steps to mindful eating

- For your mealtime, choose a calm and peaceful environment with minimal distractions.
- Before you start your meal, take a few deep breaths.
- You can take a moment to appreciate your food and its textures and presentation.
- Start eating slowly and take small bites.
- As you continue to eat, pay attention to the textures and flavors of the food.
- You can put down your utensils and pause between bites to assess how full you are.
- Pause to sip water and non-caffeinated beverages.
- Your mind can wander or become distracted quickly. Refocus your attention on the food in front.
- After you have finished eating, take some time to reflect on your experience. Note any emotions or sensations that may have arisen during the meal.
- Be grateful for the nourishment and sustenance that you receive from the meal.

Mindful eating can help you be more in touch with your body's hunger and fullness cues. It will also reduce your chances of binging or overeating. By practicing mindful eating, you can also improve your enjoyment of food and your vagus nerve quality.

Prebiotics and Probiotics

When taken in sufficient amounts, probiotics can offer health benefits. Prebiotics are fibers that can't be digested but provide food for beneficial bacteria in your gut. Combining probiotics with prebiotics can promote healthy bacteria balance in the gut. This may positively affect the vagus nerve, overall health, and overall health.

This is a step–by–step guide on how to consume prebiotics and probiotics.

- Probiotic-rich foods are recommended: Yogurt, sauerkraut, and sauerkraut are all examples of probiotic-rich foods. Look out for products with active and live cultures.
- Include prebiotic-rich food in your diet.
- You might consider taking a probiotic supplement: If you cannot eat enough probiotic-rich food, you may want a supplement. You should look for high-quality products that contain a wide range of beneficial bacteria strains.
- Follow the recommended dosage: Refer to the recommended probiotic supplement dosage label. There are no dosage guidelines for probiotic-rich foods. However, it is recommended that you consume them regularly as part of a healthy diet.

- Be aware of any side effects. While prebiotics and probiotics are generally safe for most people (including children), some people may experience slight digestive problems such as gas or bloating. You should consult a healthcare professional if you have any concerns or experience any side effects.

How they improve the vagus nerve

Prebiotics and probiotics work together to maintain a healthy balance in the gut. This can reduce inflammation, improve digestion, and increase immune function. It may also have positive effects on the vagus nerve. Some probiotic strains have been shown directly to stimulate the vagus neuron, which can have a calming effect and reduce anxiety.

Spend time with loved ones and engage in social activities

Spending time with family and friends can help you feel better and less stressed. This can also have a positive effect on your vagus nerve function.

These are the steps to follow:

- Regular social activities should be planned with family and friends. You can go out for dinner, attend social events, or engage in hobbies with your friends.
- Engage in meaningful conversations with your loved ones. It can foster a sense of connection and intimacy that can benefit your overall well-being.

- Take part in group activities that require collaboration and communication. You can do this by playing board games or team sports.
- When interacting with your loved ones, practice active listening and empathy. This will help you build better relationships and foster trust and understanding.
- Even if you only have a text or phone call, trycommunicating with others regularly.

Vagus Nerve Benefits:

Social activities and spending time with loved ones can reduce stress and improve well-being. This can have a positive effect on the vagus nerve function. Spending time with family and friends can improve moods and decrease feelings of loneliness. This can then have a positive impact on the nervous system. Social support is beneficial for both overall health and vagus nerve function.

Exposition to Nature

The vagus nerve can be stimulated by spending time in nature, such as in a forest or near water bodies. This can lead to various health benefits, including reduced stress, better mood, and improved immune function.

You should take these steps to make the most of your nature exposure.

- You should choose a natural setting: Look for a nearby park, forest, beach, or lake. Choose an environment that is quiet, peaceful, and without distractions.

- Get involved in nature activities. Once you have found a natural area, you can start to engage in activities such as walking, swimming, birdwatching, or just sitting and watching nature.

- Unplug technology: Disconnect from your phone and other electronic devices that could distract you from the natural world. It is essential to completely immerse yourself in nature and disconnect from the world of technology.

- Your senses are what you should be focusing on. Pay attention to all the sights, sounds, and smells around you. Deepen your breaths, and let the fresh air inhale into your lungs. Listen to the sounds of water running and birds singing. Feel the textures of the leaves and sand by touching them.

- Mindfulness: In nature, remain present and not get lost in your thoughts. Mindfulness can be practiced by paying attention to your breath, senses, and surroundings.

- You should spend as much time as you can in nature. Your body will need to unwind and relax more if you stay longer.

It is believed that spending time in nature stimulates the vagus nerve. This activates the parasympathetic nervous, which promotes relaxation. Stress, anxiety, depression, and other factors can all negatively affect vagus nerve function.

Deep Pressure Touch

Deep-pressure touch refers to sensory input that uses firm pressure on the body. This is often done by hugging or using weighted blankets. This touch can have a relaxing and calming effect on the body. It may also help to improve vagus nerve function by reducing anxiety and stress levels.

Deep pressure touch:

- Find a blanket that is snug and comfortable or a partner to hug.
- Place your feet in a comfortable place.
- You can wrap the blanket around your body or hug your partner tight.
- Allow yourself to feel the pressure and relax.
- You can remain in the same position for a few seconds or up to 30 minutes.

The vagus nerve gets the benefits of deep pressure touching:

- It reduces anxiety and stress levels by stimulating the parasympathetic nervous systems.
- Oxytocin releases oxytocin, which increases feelings of calmness and relaxation.
- This may improve the quality and length of your sleep.
- It regulates the autonomic nervous system by decreasing sympathetic nervous system activity and increasing parasympathetic nervous system activity.
- This may improve digestion by decreasing gastrointestinal motility and increasing gut-brain communication.

Not all people can use hugging and weighted blankets. Before trying new wellness methods, it's a good idea to consult a healthcare professional.

Visualization Exercise

Visualization exercises allow you to use your mind's power to create mental images and scenes that evoke feelings such as calm, positivity, relaxation, and optimism. These exercises are a great tool to improve vagus nerve function. They help reduce stress and anxiety, promote well-being, and provide inner peace.

These are the steps for a visualization exercise.

- You will feel at ease in a peaceful, quiet place.
- Take a few deep, relaxing breaths. Focus on your breath. Let stress and tension melt away.
- Imagine a serene scene in your imagination. You could imagine a serene beach or a lush forest. Or any other setting that is soothing to you.
- To fully immerse yourself in this scene, use all your senses. You can see the shapes and colors around you, the sounds and smells of nature, and feel the sun and breeze on your skin.
- Relax and let go of all worries or thoughts.
- You can stay in this visualization for as long as you like.
- Slowly open your eyes when you are ready. Next, take a few deep breaths and go back to your day.

Visualization exercises can stimulate the vagus nerve and promote relaxation. They also reduce stress and anxiety. This can then help regulate heart rate, blood pressure, digestion, and other bodily functions controlled by the vagus nerve. Visualization exercises are a great way to improve vagus nerve function.

Biofeedback Training

Biofeedback uses electronic devices to monitor and give information about physiological processes within the body, such as heart rate variability (HRV), an approach called biofeedback. These physiological processes can be controlled through biofeedback training, which combines mental and physical exercises.

Step-by-Step Procedure

- You should consult a biofeedback therapist or qualified practitioner to help you navigate the process.
- To monitor your HRV or other physiological processes, you may be asked to wear electrodes or sensors on your skin.
- Through a series of exercises, you will learn how to control your HRV.
- The biofeedback device provides real-time feedback, allowing you to adapt your techniques as needed.
- You can use these techniques daily as you gain more control over your HRV.

It Helps Improve Vagus Nerve

The ability to increase HRV through biofeedback training has improved vagus nerve function. Biofeedback training can help individuals control their HRV and improve vagus nerve function. This could reduce stress, better mood, and enhance immune function. Biofeedback training can also help people manage specific symptoms related to vagus nerve dysfunction (e.g., IBS, migraines, and irritable bowel syndrome).

Pranayama

Pranayama, a yogic practice that uses different breathing techniques, is called Pranayama. Pranayama is a Sanskrit word that refers to two words: "prana," which means life force or breath, and "ayama," which means extension or expansion. Pranayama can be used to regulate your breath and promote relaxation. This may stimulate the vagus nerve.

Kumbhaka is a pranayama breathing exercise that requires breath-holding. These are the steps for performing Kumbhaka.

- Sit comfortably seated, with your spine straightening and your shoulders relaxed.
- Start by inhaling through your nose.
- For a few seconds, hold your breath and then exhale slowly through your nose.
- After exhaling all of the air, hold your breath for a few seconds and then inhale again.
- You can repeat the cycle of exhaling and inhaling for several rounds while holding your breath.

These are some of the potential benefits of pranayama breathing exercises that stimulate vagus nerves:

- Regulates breathing, which can improve heart rate variability and promote relaxation.
- This increases the oxygen supply to the brain and may reduce anxiety and depression symptoms.
- This activates the parasympathetic nervous systems, reducing stress and promoting relaxation.

- This can improve the function of the lungs and your respiratory health.

Pranayama exercises should only be performed under the supervision of a certified yoga instructor.

Humming and singing while exhaling

Humming or singing while exhaling is an easy exercise. This involves slow and deep exhalations while singing or humming. This simple exercise has been proven to activate the parasympathetic nervous systems, which regulate the body's relaxation response. It also stimulates the vagus nerve.

Steps:

- You need to find a quiet and peaceful place to concentrate on your breathing, sing, or hum without distractions.
- Sit or stand straight with your shoulders relaxed and your feet planted on the ground.
- Take deep inhalations through your nose and mouth to calm your mind and relax your body.
- Start by singing or humming a simple tune. Choose a pitch that suits your voice best. As you sing or hum, focus on your chest and throat sensations.
- Continue to hum or sing while you exhale slowly and deeply. Aim to exhale longer than you inhale to activate the parasympathetic nervous systems and stimulate the vagus nerve.
- Sing or hum for at most 3-5 minutes. If you are feeling more comfortable, go longer.

- To help you transition to your normal breathing rhythm, continue singing or humming after your song ends. Take a few deep breaths through the nose and out through the mouth.
- This exercise can be repeated as many times as you wish, including daily and whenever you feel anxious or stressed.

Benefits:

- It activates the parasympathetic nervous system and stimulates vagus nerves, reducing stress, anxiety, inflammation, and other symptoms.
- It improves breathing technique and lung capacity. This can help to reduce stress and anxiety.
- Focuses on the present moment, sound, and bodily breath sensations. This enhances mindfulness and concentration.
- It is a fun and creative way to unwind and relax.

Journaling and Practice Gratitude

Journaling or Gratitude Practice is a simple way to express gratitude for what you have. This practice may benefit your mental and physical health and improve your vagus nerve function.

Step by step:

- You will need a place to sit down or lie down in peace.
- Take a few deep, slow breaths and let your mind settle.
- Think about everything you are grateful for, including your family, friends, and health.

- Write down or say the 3-5 things you are grateful for daily. These things will be more meaningful if you are as specific as possible.
- This practice should be repeated daily, and ideally every day simultaneously.

It helps to improve the vagus nerve.

Gratitude practices have been shown to increase activity in the prefrontal cortex and dopamine production. These effects may be beneficial for stimulating the vagus nerve. Gratitude practice has also decreased anxiety and stress, which could positively affect the vagus nerve function. Focusing on positive emotions like gratitude can help shift the body to a parasympathetic mode, activating vagus nerves and promoting relaxation.

Intermittent Fasting

Intermittent fasting is a diet involving eating and fasting in alternating periods. This way of eating has many health benefits, including weight loss, better blood sugar control, and lower inflammation.

Intermittent fasting can affect the vagus nerve in several ways. It triggers a process known as autophagy. This is the body's method of cleaning out and replacing damaged cells. Researchers have suggested that autophagy may be necessaryfor nerve cell function and health. Intermittent fasting could benefit the vagus nerve's health and functionality.

Here is a step-by-step guide on how to do intermittent fasting.

- You can choose a fasting plan: There are many options for fasting. The most popular are the 16/8 (fasting for 16 hours and eating within an 8-hour window each night) and the 15:2 (generally eating for 5 consecutive days while limiting calorie intake to 500-600 cals on two non-consecutive weeks).

Gradually increase your fasting time. If intermittent fasting is new to you, it's a good idea to increase the length of your fasting periods slowly. You might begin with a 12-hour fast, then gradually increase your fasting time to 16- or 18 hours.

Keep hydrated: You must drink plenty of water during fasting.

- You should break your fast gently. Leafy greens, nuts, and lean proteins like chicken and fish are all good options.

Intermittent fasting is not for everyone. This is especially true for those with certain medical conditions, pregnancy, or nursing. Before you start any new diet or wellness program, it's a good idea to consult your healthcare professional.

CHAPTER 11:
EASY RECIPES YOU CAN TRY

The vagus nerve plays a crucial role in regulating the digestive system and maintaining a healthy stress response. In order to keep the vagus nerve functioning at its best, it's important to have a balanced and nutritious diet that includes fiber-rich foods and other ingredients that support nerve function.

In this chapter, we will be discussing some simple and easy recipes that you can try to help boost the power of your vagus nerve. These recipes are designed to be quick and easy to make, and they are also delicious and nutritious. Whether you're looking for a quick breakfast, a tasty lunch, or a hearty dinner, these recipes will help you support your vagus nerve and keep your digestive system functioning at its best.

Below is a list of basic recipes you can try to help improve the Vagus Nerve:

Blueberries and Chia Seed Pudding

Chia seeds are rich in Omega-3 adipose acids and fiber. These can stimulate the vagus nerve to ameliorate digestive health. This recipe requires the following:

- 1 mug unsweetened almond buttermilk
- 1/4 mug chia seeds
- 1 tsp vanilla excerpt

1 tbsp maple syrup or honey

1 mug fresh blueberries

Instructions

Mix the almond milk, vanilla excerpt, chia seeds, and honey in large coliseum.

Wrap the coliseum in plastic serape and place it in the refrigerator for at least four hours or overnight.

After the admixture has thickened, add the blueberries.

Serve it in a coliseum, and enjoy!

Avocado Toast and Veggie Omelet

This breakfast recipe combines protein-rich eggs with the health benefits of avocados and vegetables. Avocados contain nutrients that can help regulate the vagus nervous system, while vegetables like bell peppers, onions, and mushrooms provide additional vitamins and minerals.

Ingredients:

2 large eggs

60 grams vegetables (such as bell peppers, onions, and mushrooms)

1 tsp olive oil

1/2 ripe avocado

120 grams of bread

Instructions:

In a large bowl, beat the eggs until well mixed.

Heat the olive oil in a large skillet over medium heat.

Add the chopped vegetables to the skillet and cook for about 5 minutes, or until they are tender.

- Pour the beaten eggs into the skillet and cook until they are well-set.
- While the eggs are cooking, toast the bread until it is golden brown.
- Slice the avocado in half and remove the pit. Mash the flesh with a fork until it is smooth.
- Spread the mashed avocado on the toasted bread.
- Serve the avocado toast with the vegetable omelet.

Sweet Potato and Turkey Sausage Hash recipe

This hearty breakfast dish combines sweet potatoes and turkey sausage for a nutritious and flavorful meal. Sweet potatoes are an excellent source of potassium, which can help regulate the vagus nerve, while turkey sausage provides a good source of protein.

Ingredients:

- 300 grams of sweet potato
- 200 grams of turkey sausage
- 1 tsp olive oil
- Salt and pepper to taste

Instructions:

- Heat the olive oil in a large skillet over medium heat.
- Add the diced sweet potato to the skillet and cook for about 10 minutes, or until the sweet potatoes are tender and lightly browned.
- Add the diced turkey sausage to the skillet and continue cooking for about 5 minutes, or until the sausage is golden brown.
- Season with salt and pepper to taste.
- Serve hot.

Yogurt Parfait With Berries and Almonds

This delicious and nutritious parfait combines Greek yogurt with fresh berries and almonds for a healthy and satisfying breakfast or snack. Greek yogurt is rich in probiotics that can improve gut health and help regulate the vagus nerve.

Ingredients:

- 240 mililiters of yogurt
- 80 grams of fresh berries (such as blueberries, raspberries, and strawberries)
- 30 grams almonds
- 1 tbsp maple syrup or honey

Instructions:

- In a large bowl, mix together the Greek yogurt and maple syrup or honey until well combined.
- Layer the yogurt mixture with the fresh berries and chopped almonds in a large glass.
- Continue layering until you reach the top of the glass.
- Serve and enjoy!

Quinoa and Veggie Bowl

This healthy and tasty bowl combines quinoa and fresh vegetables for a nutritious meal that can stimulate the vagus nerve and improve digestion. Quinoa is an excellent source of fiber, which can help regulate the vagus nerve.

Ingredients:

- 200 grams cooked quinoa

- 150 grams chopped vegetables (such as bell peppers and onions)
- 1 tsp olive oil
- Salt and pepper to taste
- 30 grams feta cheese
- 1 tbsp lemon juice

Instructions:

- Heat the olive oil in a large skillet over medium heat.
- Add the chopped vegetables to the skillet and cook for about 5 minutes, or until the vegetables are tender and lightly browned.
- In a large bowl, mix together the cooked quinoa, cooked vegetables, crumbled feta cheese, and lemon juice.
- Season with salt and pepper to taste.
- Serve and enjoy!

Peanut Butter Banana Smoothie

This delicious smoothie is packed with healthy fats from peanut butter and is perfect for regulating the vagus nervous system. The recipe requires just a few simple ingredients that can be easily found in your kitchen.

Ingredients:

- 1 banana
- 240 milliliters of almond milk
- 16 grams of peanut butter
- 1 tsp honey or maple syrup
- 1 tsp vanilla extract
- Ice (optional)

Instructions:

Peel the banana and break it into chunks.

In a blender, combine the banana, unsweetened almond milk, peanut butter, honey or maple syrup, and vanilla extract.

Blend the mixture until it is smooth and creamy.

If desired, add some ice to thicken the smoothie.

Blend the mixture once again until smooth and creamy.

Pour the smoothie into a glass and enjoy!

Oatmeal with Apples & Cinnamon

Oatmeal is a great source of fiber, which can help improve digestion by stimulating the vagus nerve. This recipe requires the following ingredients:

1 cup of rolled oats

2 cups of water

1 apple, diced

1 teaspoon of ground cinnamon

1 tablespoon of honey or maple syrup

Instructions:

In a large saucepan, bring the water to a boil.

Add the rolled oats and stir well.

Reduce the heat to low and cook for about 5 minutes, stirring occasionally, until the oatmeal is tender.

Add the diced apple and ground cinnamon to the saucepan and stir well.

Cook for another 2-3 minutes until the apple is soft.

Remove from heat and stir in the honey or maple syrup.

- Serve hot and enjoy!

Turkey and Cheese Breakfast Sandwich

Turkey is a good source of protein that can help regulate vagus nerve function. This recipe requires the following:

- 2 slices whole grain bread
- 2 slices turkey
- 1 slice cheese (such as cheddar or Swiss)
- 1 egg
- Salt and pepper to your liking

Instructions:

- Toast the bread slices.
- Place the cheese and turkey on one slice of bread
- Cook the egg in a small saucepan on medium heat until it is fully cooked.
- Salt and pepper to your liking
- Add the egg to the top of the cheese, and then top it with the second piece of bread.
- Serve and enjoy

Spinach and Feta Frittata

Spinach is rich in antioxidants that can regulate the vagus nerve. This recipe requires the following:

- 1 cup spinach
- 6 eggs
- 1/4 cup feta cheese, crumbled
- 1 tsp olive oil

- Salt and pepper to your liking

Instructions:

- Over medium heat, heat the olive oil in a large saucepan.
- Cook the spinach until it is wilted for about 2 minutes.
- Beat the eggs in a large bowl and place them separately.
- Add the eggs to the pan along with the spinach.
- Sprinkle the feta cheese over it.
- Cook the eggs until they are completely set, approximately 5 minutes.
- Salt and pepper to your liking
- Serve hot

Turkey Bacon and Egg Breakfast

Turkey bacon is an excellent source of protein that can regulate the vagus nerve. This recipe requires the following:

- 4 slices of turkey bacon
- 4 eggs
- 1 avocado, sliced
- 1/4 cup cherry tomatoes, halved
- Salt and pepper to your liking

Instructions:

- Heat a large pan over medium heat.
- The turkey bacon should be cooked until crisp, approximately 5 minutes
- Cook the eggs in the same pan until you are satisfied with them.
- Combine the avocado, cherry tomatoes, and cooked bacon in a large bowl.

- Salt and pepper to your liking
- Place the eggs on top of the avocado, cherry tomatoes, and bacon.

FREQUENTLY ASKED QUESTIONS

How do you define the vagus nerve and what's the reason for its importance?

Vagus is one of the longest that runs through the body. It runs through the brainstem and into the abdomen. It plays an important role in regulating the body's responses to stress and promotes relaxation. It also plays an important role in the regulation of digestion as well as the immune system, heart rate as well as blood pressure.

Exercises for vagus nerves be risky?

Like any fitness routine, it's crucial to speak with a healthcare expert or a certified practitioner before beginning any new workout routine, particularly if suffering from any medical condition. Certain people might experience health conditions that result in certain exercises being harmful. If you feel discomfort, pain, or other signs, stop the exercise and talk to an expert in healthcare.

What is the time it will require for exercises to stimulate the vagus nerve to begin working?

It is important to keep in mind that each person's experience will be different and it could take a while before you see any improvement. It's also crucial to keep in mind that these exercises must be part of a comprehensive method of improving your overall well-being and health.

Do I have to do these exercises while working?

Yes, a lot of exercises can be performed in a quiet manner and without disrupting your work. Some exercises, like the humming exercise, can be completed at work While others, like cold exposure, will require doing at your home.

Are there any food items I shouldn't eat while doing the exercises?

As was discussed in the previous chapters, a diet that is rich in refined sugars and processed food can adversely affect the functioning of the nerve and cause stress. It's also crucial to avoid drinking alcohol and caffeine when performing these exercises. It is recommended to speak with an experienced healthcare professional or certified practitioner before making any major modifications to your eating habits.

What is the recommended frequency to perform the exercises?

It's suggested to include these exercises in your daily routine. Gradually increase the time of the exercises as you get accustomed to the routine. But, it's best to talk to a health specialist or a certified practitioner to get a personalized recommendation.

Are these exercises while breastfeeding or pregnant?

It is important to speak with an expert in healthcare or a qualified practitioner before beginning any exercise program when you are pregnant or nursing.

Do I have to do these exercises while suffering from other medical ailments?

It's essential to speak with a physician or a certified practitioner before beginning any exercise program in particular if you have any medical condition. These exercises might not be appropriate for all and your doctor will be able to advise you on which exercises are the best for you.

CONCLUSION

In the end, "Daily VagusNerve Exercises " is an informative exploration of the intricate nature of the vital nerve, as well as the different methods which can be used for stimulating it. We started by exploring the anatomical and physiological aspects of the vagus nerve. This provides readers with a better knowledge of the way this intricate nerve system functions inside the body.

We also explored a range of ways to stimulate the vagus nerve, which include yoga, deep breathing exercises cold therapy, and cardiovascular training. Each of these strategies has been tested scientifically to stimulate vagus nerves and offer many benefits to health, from decreasing inflammation and improving the health of the heart as well as improving mood and alleviating symptoms of depression and anxiety.

In this book, we've stressed the importance of taking an integrated method of activating the vagus nervous system. This means the incorporation of lifestyle changes, such as regular exercising, healthy eating, and techniques for managing stress and designing a customized vagus nerve stimulation program that is most effective for you. If you take the advice and methods within this guide and incorporate them into your routine, you will be able to unlock the potential of the vagus nerve and enhance your overall quality of life.

It's important to remember that the results might not be instantaneous and it's crucial to take your time and allow your body to adjust and react to the changes that you're making. It's important to pay attention to your body and adjust as necessary and speak with an expert in your healthcare if there are any concerns.

The book explored the many ways of stimulating the Vagus nerve, and the benefits it can bring. We've also discussed the importance of a holistic approach as well as the necessity for a customized strategy. We hope our book will not only inform you about how important the vagus nerve, is but will also help you manage your health and well-being. Vagus nerves play an essential role in the regulation of various bodily functions, ranging from digestion and heart rate as well as mental and general health. If you take the knowledge and methods throughout this guide and include them in your routine, you will be able to unlock the potential of the vagus nerve to enhance your overall health.

We'd like to express our gratitude to you for spending the time to read this book and taking part in this journey to unlock the potential of the vagus nervous system. The knowledge and strategies presented here can be a useful source for improving the overall health and wellness of your family and friends. Be sure to pay attention to your body's signals and speak to a health specialist if you are experiencing any questions. Together we can unleash the power of the vagus nerve to improve the quality of our life.